Cholesterol Cure Handbook Made Simple:

Full Guide on Everything You Need to Know Regarding Cholesterol Cure; the Dos & Don'ts & Plus Other Essential Secrets You Need to Lower It in Less than 3 Days

By

Doctor JORDAN W. GALWAY

Copyright@2020

TABLE OF CONTENTS

CHAPTER ONE

INTRODUCTION

Meaning of Cholesterol:
Cholesterol is a waxy substance your liver creates to ensure and maintain nerves and to make cell tissue as well as certain hormones. Your body additionally gets cholesterol from the food you eat. This incorporates eggs, meats, and dairy. A lot of cholesterol can be terrible for your wellbeing. Cholesterol could be good or bad; that is to say we have the ones that

are bad as well as the ones that are quite good.

Find out more as I take you through all you need to know regarding cholesterol down to its cure, how it affects your health plus how to naturally manage it as well as other alternatives, and the foods you need to consume and avoid right away. Let's quickly move on to the next chapters!

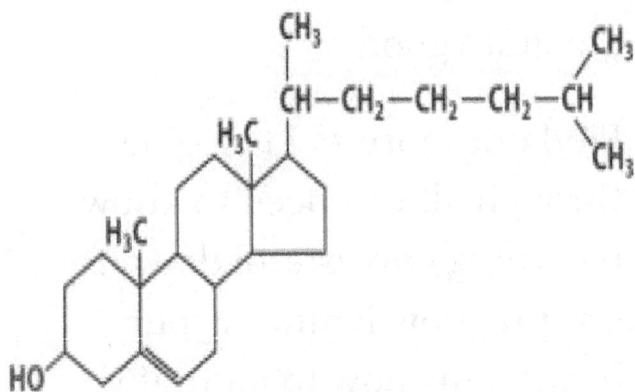

Cholesterol

CHAPTER TWO

THE COMPARISON BETWEEN GOOD AS WELL AS BAD CHOLESTEROL THAT YOU SHOULD KNOW PLUS SIGNS OF INCREASED CHOLESTEROL

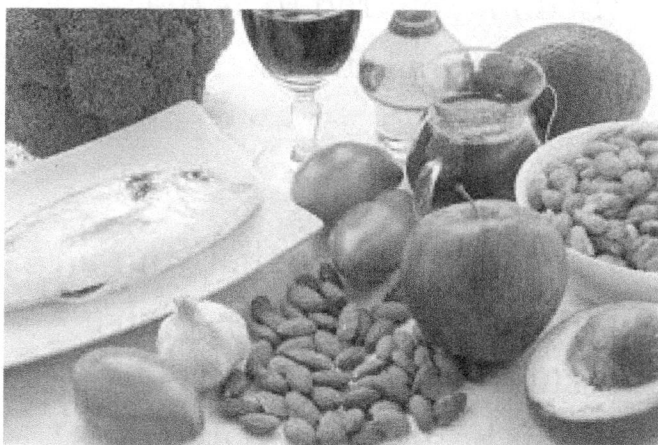

What is the comparison between "abundant" cholesterol as well "appalling" cholesterol?

Great cholesterol is known as high-thickness lipoprotein (HDL). It expels cholesterol from the circulatory system. Little-thickness lipoprotein (LDL) is referred to as the "unpleasant" cholesterol.

On the off chance that your all out cholesterol level is high a result of a high LDL level, you might be at higher danger of coronary illness or stroke. However, in the event that your complete cholesterol level is high simply because of a high HDL level, you're likely not at higher hazard.

Triglycerides are another sort of fat in your blood. At the point when you eat a bigger number of calories than your body can utilize, it transforms the additional calories into triglycerides.

Changing your way of life (diet and exercise) can improve your cholesterol levels, lower LDL and triglycerides, and raise HDL.

Your optimal cholesterol level will rely upon your hazard for coronary illness.

• Total cholesterol level – under 200 is ideal, however it relies upon your HDL and LDL levels.

- LDL cholesterol levels – under 130 is ideal, however this relies upon your hazard for coronary illness.

- HDL cholesterol levels – 60 or higher lessens your hazard for coronary illness.

- Triglycerides – under 150 milligrams for each deciliter (mg/dl) is ideal.

Manifestations of elevated cholesterol

Regularly, there are no particular side effects of elevated cholesterol. You could have elevated cholesterol and not know it.

In the event that you have elevated cholesterol, your body may store the additional cholesterol in your corridors. These are veins that convey blood from your heart to the remainder of your body. A development of cholesterol in your supply routes is known as plaque. After some time, plaque can turn out to be hard and make your corridors thin. Enormous stores of plaque can totally obstruct a vein. Cholesterol plaques can likewise break separated, prompting arrangement of a blood coagulation that obstructs the progression of blood.

A blocked supply route to the heart can cause a respiratory failure. A blocked corridor to your cerebrum can cause a stroke.

Numerous individuals don't find that they have elevated cholesterol until they endure one of these dangerous occasions. A few people discover through standard registration that incorporate blood tests.

CHAPTER THREE

AMAZING NATURAL APPROACHES TO TREAT CHOLESTEROL ISSUES

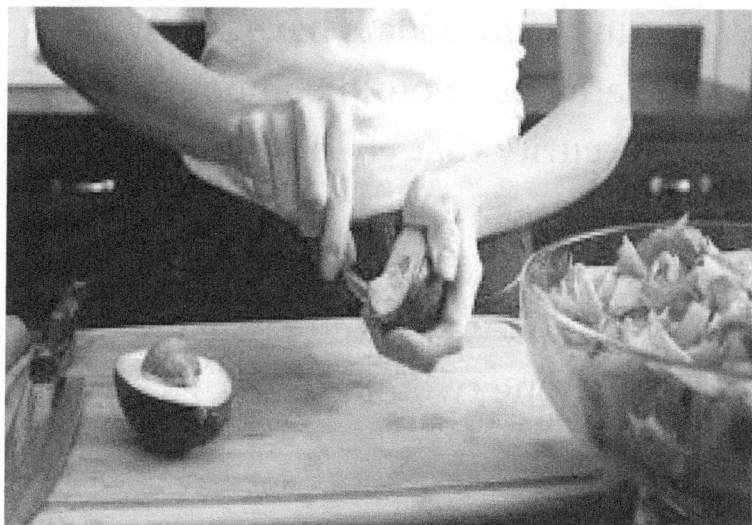

The following are 10 characteristic approaches to

improve your cholesterol levels.

1. Concentrate on Monounsaturated Fats

Rather than immersed fats, unsaturated fats have at any rate one twofold compound security that changes the manner in which they are utilized in the body. Monounsaturated fats have just one twofold security.

Albeit some suggest a low-fat eating regimen for weight reduction, an investigation of

10 men found a 6-week, low-fat eating regimen decreased degrees of destructive LDL, yet additionally diminished helpful HDL

Conversely, an eating regimen high in monounsaturated fats decreased hurtful LDL, yet additionally ensured more elevated levels of solid HDL.

An investigation of 24 grown-ups with high blood cholesterol reached a similar determination, where eating an eating routine high in monounsaturated fat expanded useful HDL by 12%, contrasted with an eating regimen low in immersed fat

Monounsaturated fats may likewise decrease the oxidation of lipoproteins, which adds to obstructed courses. An investigation of 26 individuals found that supplanting polyunsaturated fats with monounsaturated fats in the eating routine decreased the oxidation of fats and cholesterol .

Generally speaking, monounsaturated fats are solid since they decline hurtful LDL cholesterol, increment great HDL cholesterol and decrease destructive oxidation.

The following are monounsaturated fats. Some are additionally acceptable wellsprings of polyunsaturated fat include:

- Olives and olive oil

- Canola oil

• Tree nuts, for example, almonds, pecans, walnuts, hazelnuts and cashews

• Avocados

2. Utilize Polyunsaturated Fats, Especially Omega-3s

Polyunsaturated fats have various twofold securities that cause them to act distinctively in the body than immersed fats. Examination shows that polyunsaturated fats diminish "awful" LDL cholesterol and reduction the danger of coronary illness.

For instance, one examination supplanted soaked fats in 115 grown-ups' weight control plans with polyunsaturated fats for about two months. Before the end, aggregate and LDL cholesterol levels were decreased by about 10% .

Another investigation included 13,614 grown-ups. They supplanted dietary soaked fat with polyunsaturated fat, giving about 15% of complete calories. Their danger of coronary supply route infection dropped by almost 20% .

Polyunsaturated fats additionally appear to decrease the danger of metabolic condition and type 2 diabetes.

Another investigation changed the weight control plans of 4,220 grown-ups, supplanting 5% of their calories from starches with polyunsaturated fats. Their blood glucose and fasting insulin levels diminished, demonstrating a diminished danger of type 2 diabetes).

Omega-3 unsaturated fats are a particularly heart-sound kind of polyunsaturated fat. They're found in fish and fish oil supplements.

Omega-3 fats are found in high sums in greasy fish like salmon, mackerel, herring and remote ocean fish like bluefin or tuna, and less significantly in shellfish including shrimp .

Different wellsprings of omega-3s incorporate seeds and tree nuts, however not peanuts.

Summary for You

All polyunsaturated fats are heart-solid and may decrease the danger of diabetes. Omega-3 fats are a sort of polyunsaturated fat with additional heart benefits.

3. Keep away from Trans Fats

Trans fats are unsaturated fats that have been altered by a procedure called hydrogenation.

This is done to make the unsaturated fats in vegetable oils increasingly steady as a fixing. Numerous margarines and shortenings are made of somewhat hydrogenated oils.

The subsequent trans fats are not completely immersed, however are strong at room temperatures. This is the reason food organizations have utilized trans fats in items like spreads, baked goods and treats — they give more surface than unsaturated, fluid oils.

Lamentably, mostly hydrogenated trans fats are dealt with diversely in the body than different fats, and not positively. Trans fats increment all out cholesterol and LDL, however decline valuable HDL by as much as 20% .

An investigation of worldwide wellbeing designs assessed trans fats might be liable for 8% of passings from coronary illness around the world. Another investigation evaluated a law limiting trans fats in New York will diminish coronary illness passings by 4.5%.

In the United States and an expanding number of different

nations, food organizations are required to list the measure of trans fats in their items on nourishment names.

Be that as it may, these names can be deceiving, in light of the fact that they are permitted to adjust down when the measure of trans fat per serving is under 0.5 grams. This implies a few nourishments contain trans fats despite the fact that their marks state "0 grams of trans fat per serving."

To stay away from this stunt, read the fixings notwithstanding the sustenance mark. On the off chance that an item contains "in part hydrogenated" oil, it has trans fats and ought to be maintained a strategic distance from.

Summary for You

Foods with "somewhat hydrogenated" oil in the fixings contain trans fats and are hurtful, regardless of whether the mark guarantees the item has "o grams of trans fat per serving."

4. Eat/Consume Soluble Fiber

Solvent fiber is a gathering of various mixes in plants that break down in water and that people can't process.

In any case, the gainful microorganisms that live in your digestive organs can process solvent fiber. Truth be told, they require it for their own sustenance. These great microorganisms, likewise called probiotics, lessen both hurtful sorts of lipoproteins, LDL and VLDL.

In an investigation of 30 grown-ups, taking 3 grams of solvent fiber supplements day by day for 12 weeks diminished LDL by 18%.

An alternate investigation of braced breakfast oat found that additional dissolvable fiber from gelatin decreased

LDL by 4% and fiber from psyllium diminished LDL by 6%.

Dissolvable fiber can likewise help increment the cholesterol advantages of taking a statin prescription.

One 12-week study had 68 grown-ups include 15 grams of the psyllium item Metamucil to their everyday 10-mg portion of the lipid-bringing down drug simvastatin. This was seen as compelling as

taking a bigger 20-mg portion
of the statin without fiber

Dissolvable fiber's advantages
decrease the danger of
ailment. An enormous audit of
a few investigations discovered
high fiber admissions of both
solvent and insoluble fiber
decreased the danger of death
more than 17 years by almost
15%.

Another investigation of more
than 350,000 grown-ups found
those eating the most fiber
from grains and oats lived

longer, and they were 15–20% less inclined to kick the bucket during the 14-year study.

Probably the best wellsprings of dissolvable fiber incorporate beans, peas and lentils, natural product, oats and entire grains. Fiber supplements like psyllium are additionally sheltered and reasonable sources.

Summary for You

Soluble fiber supports sound probiotic gut microscopic organisms and expels cholesterol from the body, lessening LDL and VLDL. Great sources incorporate beans, peas, lentils, natural product, psyllium and entire grains including oats.

5. Exercise

Exercise is a success win for heart wellbeing. In addition to the fact that it improves physical wellness and help battle weight, yet it additionally lessens destructive LDL and increments valuable HDL .

In one investigation, twelve weeks of joined vigorous and opposition practice decreased the particularly hurtful oxidized LDL in 20 overweight ladies.

These ladies practiced three days out of every week with 15 minutes every one of vigorous action including strolling and hopping jacks, obstruction band preparing and low-force Korean move.

While even low-power practice like strolling builds HDL, making your activity longer and increasingly extraordinary expands the advantage.

In view of an audit of 13 investigations, 30 minutes of action five days seven days is sufficient to improve cholesterol and lessen the danger of coronary illness.

In a perfect world, vigorous action should raise the pulse to about 75% of its greatest. Opposition preparing ought to be half of most extreme exertion.

Movement that raises the pulse to 85% of its greatest expands HDL and furthermore diminishes LDL. The more extended the span, the more prominent the impacts

Opposition exercise can diminish LDL even at unassuming force. At greatest exertion it likewise expands HDL. Expanding the quantity of sets or redundancies builds the advantage

Summary for You

Any sort of activity improves cholesterol and advances heart wellbeing. The more extended and increasingly serious the activity, the more prominent the advantage.

6. Shed pounds

Eating less junk food impacts the manner in which your body retains and creates cholesterol.

A two-year investigation of 90 grown-ups on one of three

haphazardly relegated weight reduction eats less carbs discovered weight reduction on any of the eating regimens expanded the assimilation of cholesterol from the eating routine and diminished the making of new cholesterol in the body

Over these two years, "great" HDL expanded while "awful" LDL didn't change, in this way lessening the danger of coronary illness.

In another comparative investigation of 14 more established men, "awful" LDL diminished too, giving much more heart assurance

An investigation of 35 young ladies indicated diminished production of new cholesterol in the body during weight reduction more than a half year

In general, weight reduction has a twofold advantage on cholesterol by expanding gainful HDL and diminishing hurtful LDL.

Summary for You

Weight misfortune diminishes absolute cholesterol, to a limited extent by diminishing the making of new cholesterol in the liver. Weight reduction has had extraordinary, however for the most part valuable, impacts on HDL and LDL in various examinations.

7. Try not to Smoke

Smoking expands the danger of coronary illness in a few different ways. One of these includes making a change to how the human body takes care of cholesterol.

The resistant cells in smokers can't return cholesterol from vessel dividers to the blood for transport to the liver. This harm is identified with tobacco tar, as opposed to nicotine

These broken invulnerable cells may add to the quicker

advancement of obstructed supply routes in smokers.

In a huge investigation of a few thousand grown-ups in Pacific Asia, smoking was related with diminished HDL levels and expanded all out cholesterol

Luckily, quitting any pretense of smoking can switch these destructive impacts.

Summary for You

Smoking seems to expand awful lipoproteins, decline "great" HDL and ruin the body's capacity to send cholesterol back to the liver to be put away or separated. Stopping smoking can invert these impacts.

8. Use Alcohol in Moderation

At the point when utilized with some restraint, the ethanol in mixed beverages

builds HDL and diminishes
the danger of coronary illness.

An investigation of 18 grown-
up ladies found that drinking
24 grams of liquor from white
wine day by day improved
HDL by 5%, contrasted with
drinking equivalent measures
of white grape juice

Liquor additionally improves
"invert cholesterol transport,"
which means cholesterol is
expelled from blood and vessel
dividers and reclaimed to the

liver. This decreases the danger of stopped up corridors and coronary illness

While moderate liquor admission decreases coronary illness chance, an excessive amount of liquor hurts the liver and builds the danger of reliance. As far as possible is two beverages every day for men and one for ladies

Summary for You

Beverages for each day may improve HDL cholesterol and decrease the danger of obstructed corridors. Be that as it may, heavier liquor use builds coronary illness hazard and damages the liver.

9. Consider Plant Sterols and Stanols

Different kinds of enhancements show guarantee for overseeing cholesterol.

Plant stanols and sterols are plant adaptations of cholesterol. Since they look like cholesterol, they are ingested from the eating routine like cholesterol.

In any case, since parts of their science are unique in relation to human cholesterol, they don't add to stopped up courses.

Rather, they lessen cholesterol levels by contending with human cholesterol. At the point when plant sterols are assimilated from the eating routine, this replaces the retention of cholesterol.

Limited quantities of plant stanols and sterols are normally found in vegetable oils, and are additionally added to specific oils and spread substitutes.

One investigation of 60 people discovered devouring yogurt with one gram of plant stanols decreased LDL by about 15%, contrasted with a fake treatment. Another examination demonstrated they diminished LDL by 20%

Regardless of these advantages to cholesterol, accessible investigations have not demonstrated that stanols or sterols decline the danger of coronary illness. The higher portions in supplements are not also tried as the little dosages in vegetable oils.

Summary for You

Plant stanols and sterols in vegetable oil or margarines contend with cholesterol ingestion and diminish LDL by up to 20%. They are not demonstrated to decrease coronary illness.

10. Attempt Supplements

There is solid proof that fish oil and solvent fiber improve cholesterol and advance heart wellbeing. Another enhancement, coenzyme Q10, is indicating guarantee in improving cholesterol, despite the fact that its drawn out advantages are not yet known.

Fish Oil

Fish oil is wealthy in the omega-3 unsaturated fats docosahexaenoic corrosive (DHA) and eicosapentaenoic corrosive (EPA).

One investigation of 42 grown-ups found that taking 4 grams of fish oil day by day diminished the aggregate sum of fat being conveyed in blood. In another investigation, taking 6 grams of fish oil every day expanded HDL

An investigation of more than 15,000 grown-ups likewise found that omega-3 unsaturated fats, including from fish oil supplements, decreased the danger of coronary illness and delayed future

Psyllium

Psyllium is a type of solvent fiber accessible as an enhancement.

A four-week investigation of 33 grown-ups found that treats enhanced with 8 grams of psyllium diminished absolute cholesterol and LDL cholesterol by almost 10%

Another examination discovered comparative outcomes utilizing a 5-gram psyllium supplement twice every day. LDL and all out cholesterol diminished by about 5% over a more drawn out, 26-week time frame

Coenzyme Q10

Coenzyme Q10 is a food substance that assists cells with delivering vitality. It is like a nutrient, then again, actually the body can create its own Q10, forestalling inadequacy.

Regardless of whether there is no insufficiency, extra Q10 as enhancements may have benefits in certain circumstances.

A few examinations with a sum of 409 members discovered coenzyme Q10 supplements decreased all out cholesterol. In these investigations, LDL and HDL didn't change

Coenzyme Q10 enhancements may likewise be gainful in rewarding cardiovascular breakdown, however it's indistinct whether they lessen the danger of creating cardiovascular breakdown or coronary failures

Summary for You

Fish oil supplements and dissolvable fiber supplements like psyllium improve cholesterol and decrease the danger of coronary illness. Coenzyme Q10 supplements diminish all out cholesterol levels, yet it's indistinct whether this forestalls coronary illness.

CHAPTER FOUR

THE CONNECTION BETWEEEN DIETARY AS WELL AS BLOOD CHOLESTEROL

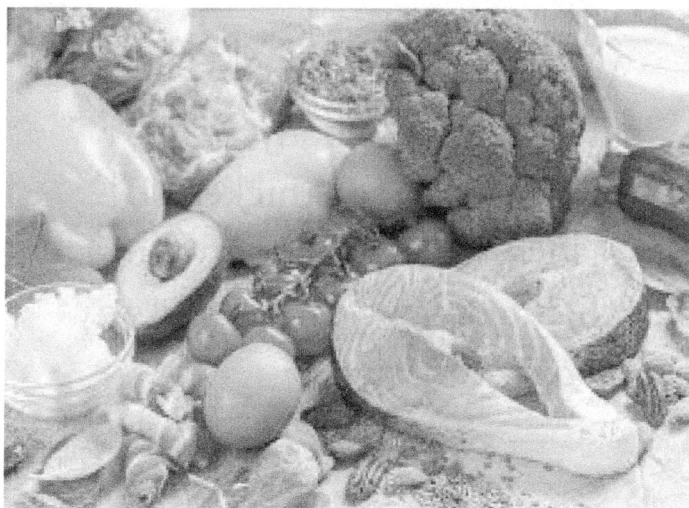

The liver does the production of adequate cholesterol the body needs. It bundles cholesterol with fat in low-thickness lipoproteins (VLDL).

As VLDL conveys fat to cells all through the body, it changes into the thicker LDL, or low-thickness lipoprotein, which conveys cholesterol any place it is required.

The liver additionally discharges high-thickness lipoprotein (HDL), which conveys unused cholesterol back to the liver. This procedure is called switch cholesterol transport, and secures against stopped up courses and different kinds of coronary illness.

A few lipoproteins, particularly LDL and VLDL, are inclined to harm by free radicals in a procedure called oxidation. Oxidized LDL and VLDL are much progressively destructive to heart wellbeing

Despite the fact that food organizations regularly promote items as low in cholesterol, dietary cholesterol in reality just affects the measure of cholesterol in the body.

This is on the grounds that the liver changes the measure of cholesterol it makes relying upon the amount you eat. At the point when your body assimilates more cholesterol from your eating regimen, it makes less in the liver.

For instance, an examination haphazardly appointed 45 grown-ups to eat more cholesterol as two eggs day by day. At long last, those eating more cholesterol didn't have higher complete cholesterol levels or changes in lipoproteins, contrasted with those eating less cholesterol.

While dietary cholesterol has little effect on cholesterol

levels, different nourishments in your eating regimen can decline them, as can family ancestry, smoking and a stationary way of life.

Moreover, a few other way of life decisions can help increment the gainful HDL and reduction the destructive LDL.

CHAPTER FIVE

MORE ON CHOLESTEROL MEALS THAT YOU SHOULD KNOW NOW

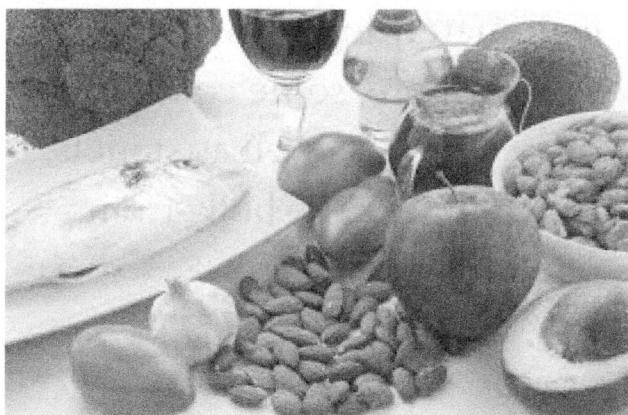

Add these nourishments to bring down LDL cholesterol

Various nourishments lower cholesterol in different manners. Some give you polyunsaturated fats, which legitimately lower LDL. Furthermore, some contain plant sterols as well as stanols, which hinder the body from retaining cholesterol.

1. Oats. A simple initial step to bringing down your cholesterol is having a bowl of oats or cold oat-based grain like Cheerios for breakfast. It gives you 1 to 2 grams of dissolvable fiber. An inclusion of a banana or a bit of strawberries for different half-gram. Current sustenance rules prescribe getting 20 to 35 grams of fiber daily, with in any event 5 to 10 grams originating from dissolvable fiber. (The normal American gets about a large portion of that sum.)

2. Grain and other entire grains. Like oats and oat

wheat, grain and other entire grains can help bring down the danger of coronary illness, principally by means of the solvent fiber they convey.

3. Beans. Beans are particularly wealthy in solvent fiber. They additionally take some time for the body to process, which means you feel full for longer after a supper. That is one explanation beans are valuable nourishment for people attempting to get in shape. With such a large number of decisions — from naval force and kidney beans to lentils, garbanzos, dark peered toward peas, and past — thus numerous approaches to set them up, beans are an extremely flexible food.

4. Eggplant and okra. These two low-calorie vegetables are acceptable wellsprings of dissolvable fiber.

5. Nuts. A bushel of studies shows that eating almonds, pecans, peanuts, and different nuts is useful for the heart.

Eating 2 ounces of nuts a day can somewhat bring down LDL, on the request for 5%. Nuts have extra supplements that secure the heart in different manners.

6. Vegetable oils. Utilizing fluid vegetable oils, for example, canola, sunflower, safflower, and others instead of margarine, fat, or shortening when cooking or at the table help lower LDL.

7. Apples, grapes, strawberries, citrus organic products. These organic products are wealthy in gelatin, a kind of solvent fiber that brings down LDL.

8. Nourishments sustained with sterols and stanols. Sterols and stanols removed from plants gum up the body's capacity to ingest cholesterol from food. Organizations are adding them to nourishments running from margarine and granola bars to squeezed orange and chocolate. They're additionally accessible as enhancements. Make handle two grams of sterols (plant) or stanols daily can balance LDL cholesterol by an amount of about 10%.

9. Soy. Eating soybeans and nourishments produced using them, similar to tofu and soy milk was once touted as an amazing method to bring down cholesterol. Investigations show that the impact is progressively unobtrusive — devouring 25 grams of soy protein daily (10 ounces of tofu or 2 1/2 cups of soy milk) can bring down LDL by 5% to 6%.

10. Greasy fish. Eating fish a few times each week can bring down LDL in two different ways: by supplanting meat, which has LDL-boosting immersed fats, and by conveying LDL-bringing down omega-3 fats. Omega-3s diminish triglycerides in the circulation system and furthermore ensure the heart by forestalling the beginning of irregular heart rhythms.

11. Fiber supplements (More explanation)

Two teaspoons every day of psyllium, which is found in Metamucil and other mass shaping intestinal medicines, give around 4 grams of dissolvable fiber.

Assembling a low cholesterol diet

With regards to putting away cash, specialists suggest making an arrangement of various speculations as opposed to tying up your assets in one place. Similar remains same for your very eating approach to balance cholesterol reasonably. Adding a few nourishments to bring down cholesterol in various manners should work superior to concentrating on a couple.

A to a great extent veggie lover "dietary arrangement of cholesterol-bringing down nourishments" considerably brings down LDL, triglycerides, and circulatory strain. The key dietary parts are a lot of products of the soil, entire grains rather than exceptionally refined ones, and protein for the most part from plants. Include margarine improved with plant sterols; oats, grain, psyllium, okra, and eggplant, all wealthy in dissolvable fiber; soy protein; and entire almonds.

Obviously, moving to a cholesterol-bringing down eating routine takes more consideration than popping an everyday statin. It implies growing the assortment of nourishments you for the most part put in your shopping basket and becoming accustomed to new surfaces and flavors. In any case, it's a "characteristic" approach to bring down cholesterol, and it keeps away from the danger of muscle issues and opposite reactions that plague a few people who take statins.

Similarly as significant, an eating routine that is substantial on organic products, vegetables, beans, and nuts is useful for the body in manners past bringing down cholesterol. It holds circulatory strain within proper limits. It assists conduits with remaining adaptable and responsive. It's useful for bones and stomach related wellbeing, for vision and emotional well-being.

CHAPTER SIX

CONCLUSION

Cholesterol care vital importance in the body yet can cause immobile supply routes and coronary illness when it gains out of power.

Low-thickness lipoprotein (LDL) is inclined to free extreme harm and contributes most to coronary illness. Interestingly, high-thickness lipoprotein (HDL) secures against coronary illness via diverting cholesterol from vessel dividers and back to the liver.

In the event that your cholesterol is out of equalization, ways of life intercessions are the main line of treatment.

Unsaturated fats, dissolvable fiber and plant sterols and stanols can expand great HDL and lessening awful LDL. Exercise and weight reduction can likewise help.

Eating trans fats and smoking is hurtful and ought to be maintained at a strategic distance from you.

In case you're worried about your cholesterol levels, have them checked by your primary care physician. A basic blood draw, taken after a short-term is quite required.

Lastly, to get the expected results, it is advisable you seriously follow the guidelines

explained in this amazing
guide!

THE END

Made in the USA
Monee, IL
28 December 2024

75559345R00049